All You Need to Know About Cancer

Learn About Cancer Etiology, Clinical Signs and Symptoms, Prevention, and Treatment.

Keith Garner , M.D

Contents

INTRODUCTION

Millions of People around the world are living with a diagnosis of cancer. This book is a gold mine of information on cancer. You will learn about possible causes, screening tests, symptoms, diagnosis, and treatment. You will also learn about proven coping mechanisms for people living with cancer.

Researchers are learning more about what causes cancer, and how it grows and progresses. And they are looking for new and better ways to prevent, detect, and treat it. Researchers also are looking for ways to improve the quality of life for people with cancer during and after their treatment.

CHAPTER ONE

UNDERSTANDING CANCER

Cancer begins in cells, the building blocks that form tissues. Tissues make up the organs of the body.

Normally, cells grow and divide to form new cells as the body needs them. When cells grow old, they die, and new cells take their place.

Sometimes, this orderly process goes wrong. New cells form when the body does not need them, and old cells do not die when they should. These extra cells can form a mass of tissue called a growth or tumor.

TUMORS CAN BE BENIGN OR MALIGNANT:

• Benign tumors are not cancer:

—Benign tumors are rarely life-threatening.

—Generally, benign tumors can be removed, and they usually do not grow back.

—Cells from benign tumors do not invade the tissues around them.

—Cells from benign tumors do not spread to other parts of the body.

• Malignant tumors are cancer:

—Malignant tumors are generally more serious than benign tumors. They may be life-threatening.

—Malignant tumors often can be removed, but sometimes they grow back.

—Cells from malignant tumors can invade and damage nearby tissues and organs.

—Cells from malignant tumors can spread (metastasize) to other parts of the body. Cancer cells spread by breaking away from the original (primary) tumor and entering the bloodstream or lymphatic system. The cells can invade other organs, forming new tumors that damage these organs. The spread of cancer is called metastasis.

Most cancers are named for where they start. For example, lung cancer starts in the lung, and breast cancer starts in the breast. Lymphoma is cancer that starts in the lymphatic system, and leukemia is cancer that starts in the white blood cells (leukocytes).

When cancer spreads and forms a new tumor in another part of the body, the new tumor has the same kind of abnormal cells and the same name as the primary tumor. For example, if prostate cancer spreads to the bones, the cancer cells in the bones are actually prostate cancer cells. The disease is metastatic prostate cancer, not bone cancer. For that reason, it is treated as prostate cancer, not bone cancer. Doctors sometimes call the new tumor "distant" or metastatic disease.

RISK FACTORS

Doctors often cannot explain why one person develops cancer and another does not. But research shows that certain risk factors increase the chance that a person will develop cancer. These are the most common risk factors for cancer:

• Growing older

• Tobacco

• Sunlight

• Ionizing radiation

• Certain chemicals and other substances

• Some viruses and bacteria

• Certain hormones

• Family history of cancer

• Alcohol

• Poor diet, lack of physical activity, or being overweight

Many of these risk factors can be avoided. Others, such as family history, cannot be avoided. People can help protect themselves by staying away from known risk factors whenever possible.

If you think you may be at risk for cancer, you should discuss this concern with your doctor. You may want to ask about reducing your risk and about a schedule for checkups.

Over time, several factors may act together to cause normal cells to become cancerous. When thinking about your risk of getting cancer, these are some things to keep in mind:

• Not everything causes cancer.

• Cancer is not caused by an injury, such as a bump or bruise.

• Cancer is not contagious. Although being infected with certain viruses or bacteria may increase the risk of some types of cancer, no one can "catch" cancer from another person.

• Having one or more risk factors does not mean that you will get cancer. Most people who have risk factors never develop cancer.

• Some people are more sensitive than others to the known risk factors.

The sections below have more detailed information about the most common risk factors for cancer.

GROWING OLDER

The most important risk factor for cancer is growing older. Most cancers occur in people over the age of 65. But people of all ages, including children, can get cancer, too.

TOBACCO

Tobacco use is the most preventable cause of death.

Each year, more than 180,000 Americans die from cancer that is related to tobacco use. Using tobacco products or regularly being around tobacco smoke (environmental or secondhand smoke) increases the risk of cancer.

Smokers are more likely than nonsmokers to develop cancer of the lung, larynx (voice box), mouth, esophagus, bladder, kidney, throat, stomach, pancreas, or cervix. They also are more likely to develop acute myeloid leukemia (cancer that starts in blood cells).

People who use smokeless tobacco (snuff or chewing tobacco) are at increased risk of cancer of the mouth.

SUNLIGHT

Ultraviolet (UV) radiation comes from the sun, sunlamps, and tanning booths. It causes early aging of the skin and skin damage that can lead to skin cancer.

Doctors encourage people of all ages to limit their time in the sun and to avoid other sources of UV radiation:

• It is best to avoid the midday sun (from mid- morning to late afternoon) whenever possible. You also should protect yourself from UV radiation reflected by sand, water, snow, and ice. UV radiation can penetrate light clothing, windshields, and windows.

• Wear long sleeves, long pants, a hat with a wide brim, and sunglasses with lenses that absorb UV.

• Use sunscreen. Sunscreen may help prevent skin cancer, especially sunscreen with a sun protection factor (SPF) of at least 15. But sunscreens cannot replace avoiding the sun and wearing clothing to protect the skin.

• Stay away from sunlamps and tanning booths. They are no safer than sunlight.

IONIZING RADIATION

Ionizing radiation can cause cell damage that leads to cancer. This kind of radiation comes from rays that enter the Earth's atmosphere from outer space, radioactive fallout, radon gas, x-rays, and other sources.

Radioactive fallout can come from accidents at nuclear power plants or from the production, testing, or use of atomic weapons. People exposed to fallout may have an increased risk of cancer, especially leukemia and cancers of the thyroid, breast, lung, and stomach.

Radon is a radioactive gas that you cannot see, smell, or taste. It forms in soil and rocks. People who work in mines may be exposed to radon. In some parts of the country, radon is found in houses. People exposed to radon are at increased risk of lung cancer.

Medical procedures are a common source of radiation:

• Doctors use radiation (low-dose x-rays) to take pictures of the inside of the body. These pictures help to diagnose broken bones and other problems.

• Doctors use radiation therapy (high-dose radiation from large machines or from radioactive substances) to treat cancer.

The risk of cancer from low-dose x-rays is extremely small. The risk from radiation therapy is slightly higher. For both, the benefit nearly always outweighs the small risk.

You should talk with your doctor if you are concerned that you may be at risk of cancer due to radiation.

If you live in a part of the country that has radon, you may wish to test your home for high levels of the gas. The home radon test is easy to use and inexpensive. Most hardware stores sell the test kit.

You should talk with your doctor or dentist about the need for each x-ray. You should also ask about shields to protect parts of the body that are not in the picture.

Cancer patients may want to talk with their doctor about how radiation treatment could increase their risk of a second cancer later on.

CERTAIN CHEMICALS AND OTHER SUBSTANCES

People who have certain jobs (such as painters, construction workers, and those in the chemical industry) have an increased risk of cancer. Many studies have shown that exposure to asbestos, benzene, benzidine, cadmium, nickel, or vinyl chloride in the workplace can cause cancer.

Follow instructions and safety tips to avoid or reduce contact with harmful substances both at work and at home. Although the risk is highest for workers with years of exposure, it makes sense to be careful at home when handling pesticides, used engine oil, paint, solvents, and other chemicals.

SOME VIRUSES AND BACTERIA

Being infected with certain viruses or bacteria may increase the risk of developing cancer:

• Human papillomaviruses (HPVs): HPV infection is the main cause of cervical cancer. It also may be a risk factor for other types of cancer.

• Hepatitis B and hepatitis C viruses: Liver cancer can develop after many years of infection with hepatitis B or hepatitis C.

• Human T-cell leukemia/lymphoma virus (HTLV–1): Infection with HTLV–1 increases a person's risk of lymphoma and leukemia.

• Human immunodeficiency virus (HIV): HIV is the virus that causes AIDS. People who have HIV infection are at greater risk of cancer, such as lymphoma and a rare cancer called Kaposi's sarcoma.

• Epstein-Barr virus (EBV): Infection with EBV has been linked to an increased risk of lymphoma.

• Human herpesvirus 8 (HHV8): This virus is a risk factor for Kaposi's sarcoma.

• Helicobacter pylori: This bacterium can cause stomach ulcers. It also can cause stomach cancer and lymphoma in the stomach lining.

Do not have unprotected sex or share needles. You can get an HPV infection by having sex with someone who is infected. You can get hepatitis B, hepatitis C, or HIV infection from having unprotected sex or sharing needles with someone who is infected.

You may want to consider getting the vaccine that prevents hepatitis B infection. Health care workers and others who come into contact with other people's blood should ask their doctor about this vaccine.

If you think you may be at risk for HIV or hepatitis infection, ask your doctor about being tested. These infections may not cause symptoms, but blood tests can show whether the virus is present. If so, the doctor may suggest treatment. Also, the doctor can tell you how to avoid infecting other people.

If you have stomach problems, see a doctor.

Infection with H. pylori can be detected and treated.

CERTAIN HORMONES

Doctors may recommend hormones (estrogen alone or estrogen along with progestin) to help control problems (such as hot flashes, vaginal dryness, and thinning bones) that may occur during menopause.

However, studies show that menopausal hormone therapy can cause serious side effects. Hormones may increase the risk of breast cancer, heart attack, stroke, or blood clots.

Diethylstilbestrol (DES), a form of estrogen, was given to some pregnant women in the United States between about 1940 and 1971. Women who took DES during pregnancy may have a slightly higher risk of developing breast cancer. Their daughters have an increased risk of developing a rare type of cancer of the cervix. The possible effects on their sons are under study.

FAMILY HISTORY OF CANCER

Most cancers develop because of changes (mutations) in genes. A normal cell may become a cancer cell after a series of gene changes occur.

Tobacco use, certain viruses, or other factors in a person's lifestyle or environment can cause such changes in some types of cells.

Some gene changes that increase the risk of cancer are passed from parent to child. These changes are present at birth in all cells of the body.

It is uncommon for cancer to run in a family.

However, certain types of cancer do occur more often in some families than in the rest of the population. For example, melanoma and cancers of the breast, ovary, prostate, and colon sometimes run in families. Several cases of the same cancer type in a family may be linked to inherited gene changes, which may increase the chance of developing cancers. However, environmental factors may also be involved. Most of the time, multiple cases of cancer in a family are just a matter of chance.

Alcohol

Having more than two drinks each day for many years may increase the chance of developing cancers of the mouth, throat, esophagus, larynx, liver, and breast. The risk increases with the amount of alcohol that a person drinks. For most of these cancers, the risk is higher for a drinker who uses tobacco.

Poor Diet, Lack Of Physical Activity, Or Being Overweight

People who have a poor diet, do not have enough physical activity, or are overweight may be at increased risk of several types of cancer. For example, studies suggest that people whose diet is high in fat have an increased risk of cancers of the colon, uterus, and prostate. Lack of physical activity and being overweight are risk factors for cancers of the breast, colon, esophagus, kidney, and uterus.

Having a healthy diet, being physically active, and maintaining a healthy weight may help reduce cancer risk. Doctors suggest the following:

• Eat well: A healthy diet includes plenty of foods that are high in fiber, vitamins, and minerals. This includes whole-grain breads and cereals and 5 to 9 servings of fruits and vegetables every day. Also, a healthy diet means limiting foods high in fat (such as butter, whole milk, fried foods, and red meat).

• Be active and maintain a healthy weight: Physical activity can help control your weight and reduce body fat. Most scientists agree that it is a good idea for an adult to have moderate physical activity (such as brisk walking) for at least 30 minutes on 5 or more days each week.

CHAPTER TWO

SCREENING

Some types of cancer can be found before they cause symptoms. Checking for cancer (or for conditions that may lead to cancer) in people who have no symptoms is called screening.

Screening can help doctors find and treat some types of cancer early. Generally, cancer treatment is more effective when the disease is found early.

Screening tests are used widely to check for cancers of the breast, cervix, colon, and rectum:

• Breast: A mammogram is the best tool doctors have to find breast cancer early. A mammogram is a picture of the breast made with x-rays. The NCI recommends that women in their forties and older have mammograms every 1 to 2 years. Women who are at higher-than-average risk of breast cancer should talk with their health care provider about whether to have mammograms before age 40 and how often to have them.

• Cervix: The Pap test (sometimes called Pap smear) is used to check cells from the cervix. The doctor scrapes a sample of cells from the cervix. A lab checks the cells for cancer or changes that may lead to cancer (including changes caused by human papillomavirus, the most important risk factor for cancer of the cervix). Women should begin having Pap tests 3 years after they begin having sexual intercourse, or when they reach age 21 (whichever comes first). Most women should have a Pap test at least once every 3 years.

• Colon and rectum: A number of screening tests are used to detect polyps (growths), cancer, or other problems in the colon and rectum. People aged 50 and older should be screened. People who have a higher-than-average risk of cancer of the colon or rectum should talk with their doctor about whether to have screening tests before age 50 and how often to have them.

—Fecal occult blood test: Sometimes cancer or polyps bleed. This test can detect tiny amounts of blood in the stool.

—Sigmoidoscopy: The doctor checks inside the rectum and lower part of the colon with a lighted tube called a sigmoidoscope. The doctor can usually remove polyps through the tube.

—Colonoscopy: The doctor examines inside the rectum and entire colon using a long, lighted tube called a colonoscope. The doctor can usually remove polyps through the tube.

—Double-contrast barium enema: This procedure involves several x-rays of the colon and rectum. The patient is given an enema with a barium solution, and air is pumped into the rectum. The barium and air improve the x-ray images of the colon and rectum.

—Digital rectal exam: A rectal exam is often part of a routine physical exam. The health care provider inserts a lubricated, gloved finger into the rectum to feel for abnormal areas. A digital rectal exam allows for examination of only the lowest part of the rectum.

You may have heard about other tests to check for cancer in other parts of the body. At this time, we do not know whether routine screening with these other tests saves lives. The NCI is supporting research to learn more about screening for cancers of the breast, cervix, colon, lung, ovary, prostate, and skin.

Doctors consider many factors before they suggest a screening test. They weigh factors related to the test and to the cancer that the test can detect. They also pay special attention to a person's risk for developing certain types of cancer. For example, doctors think about the person's age, medical history, general health, family history, and lifestyle. They consider how accurate the test is. In addition, doctors keep in mind the possible harms of the screening test itself. They also look at the risk of follow-up tests or surgery that the person might need to see if an abnormal test result means cancer. Doctors also think about the risks and benefits of treatment if testing finds cancer. They consider how well the treatment works and what side effects it causes.

You may want to talk with your doctor about the possible benefits and harms of being checked for cancer. The decision to be screened, like many other medical decisions, is a personal one. Each person should decide after learning about the pros and cons of screening.

CHAPTER THREE

SYMPTOMS, DIAGNOSIS AND STAGING

Cancer can cause many different symptoms. These include:

• A thickening or lump in the breast or any other part of the body

• A new mole or a change in an existing mole

• A sore that does not heal

• Hoarseness or a cough that does not go away

• Changes in bowel or bladder habits

• Discomfort after eating

• A hard time swallowing

• Weight gain or loss with no known reason

• Unusual bleeding or discharge

• Feeling weak or very tired

Most often, these symptoms are not due to cancer. They may also be caused by benign tumors or other problems. Only a doctor can tell for sure.

Anyone with these symptoms or other changes in health should see a doctor to diagnose and treat problems as early as possible.

Usually, early cancer does not cause pain. If you have symptoms, do not wait to feel pain before seeing a doctor.

DIAGNOSIS

If you have a symptom or your screening test result suggests cancer, the doctor must find out whether it is due to cancer or to some other cause. The doctor may ask about your personal and family medical history and do a physical exam. The doctor may also order lab tests, x-rays, or other tests or procedures.

LAB TESTS

Tests of the blood, urine, or other fluids can help doctors make a diagnosis. These tests can show how well an organ (such as the kidney) is doing its job. Also, high amounts of some substances may be a sign of cancer. These substances are often called tumor markers. However, abnormal lab results are not a sure sign of cancer. Doctors cannot rely on lab tests alone to diagnose cancer.

IMAGING PROCEDURES

Imaging procedures create pictures of areas inside your body that help the doctor see whether a tumor is present. These pictures can be made in several ways:

• X-rays: X-rays are the most common way to view organs and bones inside the body.

• CT scan: An x-ray machine linked to a computer takes a series of detailed pictures of your organs. You may receive a contrast material (such as dye) to make these pictures easier to read.

• Radionuclide scan: You receive an injection of a small amount of radioactive material. It flows through your bloodstream and collects in certain bones or organs. A machine called a scanner detects and measures the radioactivity. The scanner creates pictures of bones or organs on a computer screen or on film. Your body gets rid of the radioactive substance quickly.

• Ultrasound: An ultrasound device sends out sound waves that people cannot hear. The waves bounce off tissues inside your body like an echo. A computer uses these echoes to create a picture called a sonogram.

• MRI: A strong magnet linked to a computer is used to make detailed pictures of areas in your body. Your doctor can view these pictures on a monitor and can print them on film.

• PET scan: You receive an injection of a small amount of radioactive material. A machine makes pictures that show chemical activities in the body. Cancer cells sometimes show up as areas of high activity.

BIOPSY

In most cases, doctors need to do a biopsy to make a diagnosis of cancer. For a biopsy, the doctor removes a sample of tissue and sends it to a lab. A pathologist looks at the tissue under a microscope. The sample may be removed in several ways:

• With a needle: The doctor uses a needle to withdraw tissue or fluid.

• With an endoscope: The doctor uses a thin, lighted tube (an endoscope) to look at areas inside the body. The doctor can remove tissue or cells through the tube.

• With surgery: Surgery may be excisional or incisional.

—In an excisional biopsy, the surgeon removes the entire tumor. Often some of the normal tissue around the tumor is also removed.

—In an incisional biopsy, the surgeon removes just part of the tumor.

STAGING

To plan the best treatment for cancer, the doctor needs to know the extent (stage) of your disease.

For most cancers (such as breast, lung, prostate, or colon cancer), the stage is based on the size of the tumor and whether the cancer has spread to lymph nodes or other parts of the body. The doctor may order x-rays, lab tests, and other tests or procedures to learn the extent of the disease.

CHAPTER FOUR

TREATMENT

Many people with cancer want to take an active part in making decisions about their medical care. It is natural to want to learn all you can about your disease and treatment choices. However, shock and stress after the diagnosis can make it hard to think of everything you want to ask the doctor. It often helps to make a list of questions before an appointment.

To help remember what the doctor says, you may take notes or ask whether you may use a tape recorder. Some people also want to have a family member or friend with them when they talk to the doctor—to take part in the discussion, to take notes, or just to listen.

You do not need to ask all your questions at once. You will have other chances to ask the doctor or nurse to explain things that are not clear and to ask for more information.

Your doctor may refer you to a specialist, or you may ask for a referral. Specialists who treat cancer include surgeons, medical oncologists, hematologists, and radiation oncologists.

GETTING A SECOND OPINION

Before starting treatment, you may want a second opinion about your diagnosis and treatment plan. Many insurance companies will cover a second opinion if your doctor re☐uests it. It may take some time and effort to gather medical records and arrange to see another doctor. Usually it is not a problem to take several weeks to get a second opinion. In most cases, the delay in starting treatment will not make treatment less effective. But some people with cancer need treatment right away. To make sure, you should discuss this delay with your doctor.

There are a number of ways to find a doctor for a second opinion:

• Your doctor may refer you to one or more specialists. At cancer centers, several specialists often work together as a team.

• A local or state medical society, a nearby hospital, or a medical school can usually provide the names of specialists.

• The American Board of Medical Specialties (ABMS) has a list of doctors who have had training and passed exams in their specialty. You can find this list in the Official ABMS Directory of Board Certified Medical

Specialists. This directory is in most public libraries. Also, ABMS offers this information at http://www.abms.org. (Click on "Who's Certified.")

• Nonprofit organizations with an interest in cancer may be of help. See the NCI fact sheet "National Organizations That Offer Services to People With Cancer and Their Families."

TREATMENT METHODS

The treatment plan depends mainly on the type of cancer and the stage of the disease.

Doctors also consider the patient's age and general health. Often, the goal of treatment is to cure the cancer. In other cases, the goal is to control the disease or to reduce symptoms for as long as possible. The treatment plan may change over time.

Most treatment plans include surgery, radiation therapy, or chemotherapy. Some involve hormone therapy or biological therapy. In addition, stem cell transplantation may be used so that a patient can receive very high doses of chemotherapy or radiation therapy.

Some cancers respond best to a single type of treatment. Others may respond best to a combination of treatments.

Treatments may work in a specific area (local therapy) or throughout the body (systemic therapy):

• Local therapy removes or destroys cancer in just one part of the body. Surgery to remove a tumor is local therapy. Radiation to shrink or destroy a tumor also is usually local therapy.

• Systemic therapy sends drugs or substances through the bloodstream to destroy cancer cells all over the body. It kills or slows the growth of cancer cells that may have spread beyond the original tumor. Chemotherapy, hormone therapy, and biological therapy are usually systemic therapy.

Your doctor can describe your treatment choices and the expected results. You and your doctor can work together to decide on a treatment plan that is best for you.

Because cancer treatments often damage healthy cells and tissues, side effects are common. Side effects depend mainly on the type and extent of the treatment. Side effects may not be the same for each person, and they may change from one treatment session to the next.

Before treatment starts, the health care team will explain possible side effects and suggest ways to help you manage them. This team may include nurses, a dietitian, a physical therapist, and others. These include Radiation Therapy and You, Chemotherapy and You, Biological Therapy, and Eating Hints for Cancer Patients.

At any stage of cancer, supportive care is available to relieve the side effects of therapy, to control pain and other symptoms, and to ease emotional and practical problems.

You may want to ask the doctor these questions before treatment begins:

• What is my diagnosis?

• Has the cancer spread? If so, where? What is the stage of the disease?

• What is the goal of treatment? What are my treatment choices? Which do you recommend for me? Why?

• What are the expected benefits of each kind of treatment?

• What are the risks and possible side effects of each treatment? How can side effects be managed?

• Will infertility be a side effect of my treatment? Can anything be done about that? Should I consider storing sperm or eggs?

• What can I do to prepare for treatment?

• How often will I have treatments? How long will my treatment last?

• Will I have to change my normal activities? If so, for how long?

• What is the treatment likely to cost? Will my insurance cover the costs?

• What new treatments are under study? Would a clinical trial be appropriate for me?

SURGERY

In most cases, the surgeon removes the tumor and some tissue around it. Removing nearby tissue may help prevent the tumor from growing back. The surgeon may also remove some nearby lymph nodes.

The side effects of surgery depend mainly on the size and location of the tumor, and the type of operation. It takes time to heal after surgery. The time needed to recover is different for each type of surgery. It is also different for each person. It is common to feel tired or weak for a while.

Most people are uncomfortable for the first few days after surgery. However, medicine can help control the pain. Before surgery, you should discuss the plan for pain relief with the doctor or nurse. The doctor can adjust the plan if you need more pain relief.

Some people worry that having surgery (or even a biopsy) for cancer will spread the disease. This seldom happens. Surgeons use special methods and take many steps to prevent cancer cells from spreading. For example, if they must remove tissue from more than one area, they use different tools for each one. This approach helps reduce the chance that cancer cells will spread to healthy tissue.

Similarly, some people worry that exposing cancer to air during surgery will cause the disease to spread. This is not true. Air does not make cancer spread.

RADIATION THERAPY

Radiation therapy (also called radiotherapy) uses high-energy rays to kill cancer cells. Doctors use several types of radiation therapy. Some people receive a combination of treatments:

• External radiation: The radiation comes from a large machine outside the body. Most people go to a hospital or clinic for treatment 5 days a week for several weeks.

• Internal radiation (implant radiation or brachytherapy): The radiation comes from radioactive material placed in seeds, needles, or thin plastic tubes that are put in or near the tissue. The patient usually stays in the hospital. The implants generally remain in place for several days.

• Systemic radiation: The radiation comes from liquid or capsules containing radioactive material that travels throughout the body. The patient swallows the liquid or capsules or receives an injection. This type of radiation therapy can be used to treat cancer or control pain from cancer that has spread to the bone. Only a few types of cancer are currently treated in this way.

The side effects of radiation therapy depend mainly on the dose and type of radiation you receive and the part of your body that is treated. For example, radiation to your abdomen can cause nausea, vomiting, and diarrhea. Your skin in the treated area may become red, dry, and tender. You also may lose your hair in the treated area.

You may become very tired during radiation therapy, especially in the later weeks of treatment. Resting is important, but doctors usually advise patients to try to stay as active as they can.

Fortunately, most side effects go away in time. In the meantime, there are ways to reduce discomfort. If you have a side effect that is especially severe, the doctor may suggest a break in your treatment.

CHEMOTHERAPY

Chemotherapy is the use of drugs that kill cancer cells. Most patients receive chemotherapy by mouth or through a vein. Either way, the drugs enter the bloodstream and can affect cancer cells all over the body.

Chemotherapy is usually given in cycles. People receive treatment for one or more days. Then they have a recovery period of several days or weeks before the next treatment session.

Most people have their treatment in an outpatient part of the hospital, at the doctor's office, or at home. Some may need to stay in the hospital during chemotherapy.

Side effects depend mainly on the specific drugs and the dose. The drugs affect cancer cells and other cells that divide rapidly:

• Blood cells: When drugs damage healthy blood cells, you are more likely to get infections, to bruise or bleed easily, and to feel very weak and tired.

• Cells in hair roots: Chemotherapy can cause hair loss. Your hair will grow back, but it may be somewhat different in color and texture.

• Cells that line the digestive tract: Chemotherapy can cause poor appetite, nausea and vomiting, diarrhea, or mouth and lip sores.

Some drugs can affect fertility. Women may be unable to become pregnant, and men may not be able to father a child.

Although the side effects of chemotherapy can be distressing, most of them are temporary. Your doctor can usually treat or control them.

HORMONE THERAPY

Some cancers need hormones to grow. Hormone therapy keeps cancer cells from getting or using the hormones they need. It is a systemic therapy.

Hormone therapy uses drugs or surgery:

• Drugs: The doctor gives medicine that stops the production of certain hormones or prevents the hormones from working.

• Surgery: The surgeon removes organs (such as the ovaries or testicles) that make hormones.

The side effects of hormone therapy depend on the type of therapy. They include weight gain, hot flashes, nausea, and changes in fertility. In women, hormone therapy may make menstrual periods stop or become irregular and may cause vaginal dryness. In men, hormone therapy may cause impotence, loss of sexual desire, and breast growth or tenderness.

BIOLOGICAL THERAPY

Biological therapy is another type of systemic therapy. It helps the immune system (the body's natural defense system) fight cancer. For example, certain patients with bladder cancer receive BCG solution after surgery. The doctor uses a catheter to put the solution in the bladder. The solution contains live, weakened bacteria that stimulate the immune system to kill cancer cells. BCG can cause side effects. It can irritate the bladder. Some people may have nausea, a low- grade fever, or chills.

Most other types of biological therapy are given through a vein. The biological therapy travels through the bloodstream. Some people get a rash where the therapy is injected. Some have flu-like symptoms such as fever, chills, headache, muscle aches, fatigue, weakness, and nausea. Biological therapy also can cause more serious side effects, such as changes in blood pressure and breathing problems. Biological therapy is usually given at the doctor's office, clinic, or hospital.

STEM CELL TRANSPLANTATION

Transplantation of blood-forming stem cells enables patients to receive high doses of chemotherapy, radiation, or both. The high doses destroy both cancer cells and normal blood cells in the bone marrow. After the treatment, the patient receives healthy, blood- forming stem cells through a flexible tube placed in a large vein. New blood cells develop from the transplanted stem cells. Stem cells may be taken from the patient before the high-dose treatment, or they may come from another person. Patients stay in the hospital for this treatment.

The side effects of high-dose therapy and stem cell transplantation include infection and bleeding. In addition, graft-versus-host disease (GVHD) may occur in people who receive stem cells from a donor. In GVHD, the donated stem cells attack the patient's tissues. Most often, GVHD affects the liver, skin, or digestive tract. GVHD can be severe or even fatal. It can occur any time after the transplant, even years later. Drugs may help prevent, treat, or control GVHD.

CHAPTER FIVE

MISCELLENOUS INFORMATION

COMPLEMENTARY AND ALTERNATIVE MEDICINE

Some people with cancer use complementary and alternative medicine (CAM):

• An approach is generally called complementary medicine when it is used along with standard treatment.

• An approach is called alternative medicine when it is used instead of standard treatment.

Acupuncture, massage therapy, herbal products, vitamins or special diets, visualization, meditation, and spiritual healing are types of CAM.

Many people say that CAM helps them feel better. However, some types of CAM may change the way standard treatment works. These changes could be harmful. Other types of CAM could be harmful even if used alone.

Some types of CAM are expensive. Health insurance may not cover the cost.

NUTRITION AND PHYSICAL ACTIVITY

It is important for people with cancer to take care of themselves. Taking care of yourself includes eating well and staying as active as you can.

You need enough calories to maintain a good weight. You also need enough protein to keep up your strength. Eating well may help you feel better and have more energy.

Sometimes, especially during or soon after treatment, you may not feel like eating. You may be uncomfortable or tired. You may find that foods do not taste as good as they used to. In addition, the side effects of treatment (such as poor appetite, nausea, vomiting, or mouth sores) can be a problem.

Many people find they feel better when they stay active. Walking, yoga, swimming, and other activities can keep you strong and increase your energy. Exercise may reduce nausea and pain and make treatment easier to handle. It also can help relieve stress. Whatever physical activity you choose, be sure to talk to your doctor before you start. Also, if your activity causes you pain or other problems, be sure to let your doctor or nurse know about it.

FOLLOW-UP CARE

Advances in early detection and treatment mean that many people with cancer are cured. But doctors can never be certain that the cancer will not come back. Undetected cancer cells can remain in the body after treatment. Although the cancer seems to be completely removed or destroyed, it can return.

Doctors call this a recurrence.

To find out whether the cancer has returned, your doctor may do a physical exam and order lab tests, x-rays, and other tests. If you have a recurrence, you and your doctor will decide on new treatment goals and a new treatment plan.

During follow-up exams, the doctor also checks for other problems, such as side effects from cancer therapy that can arise long after treatment. Checkups help ensure that changes in health are noted and treated if needed. Between scheduled visits, you should contact the doctor if any health problems occur.

DICTIONARY

Acupuncture (AK-yoo-PUNK-cher): The technique of inserting thin needles through the skin at specific points on the body to control pain and other symptoms. It is a type of complementary and alternative medicine.

AIDS: Acquired immunodeficiency syndrome (ah-KWY-erd im-YOON-o-de-FISH-en-see SIN-drome). A disease caused by the human

Immunodeficiency virus (HIV). People with AIDS are at an increased risk for developing certain cancers and for infections that usually occur only in individuals with a weak immune system.

Bacteria (bak-TEER-ee-uh): A large group of single- cell microorganisms. Some cause infections and disease in animals and humans. The singular of bacteria is bacterium.

BCG solution: A form of biological therapy for superficial bladder cancer. A catheter is used to place the BCG solution into the bladder. The solution contains live, weakened bacteria (bacille Calmette- Guérin) that activate the immune system. The BCG solution used for bladder cancer is not the same thing as BCG vaccine, a vaccine for tuberculosis.

Benign (beh-NINE): Not cancerous. Benign tumors do not spread to tissues around them or to other parts of the body.

Biological therapy (by-o-LAHJ-i-kul): Treatment to stimulate or restore the ability of the immune system to fight infections and other diseases. Also used to lessen certain side effects that may be caused by cancer treatment. Also known as immunotherapy, biotherapy, or biological response modifier (BRM) therapy.

Biopsy (BY-op-see): The removal of cells or tissues for examination by a pathologist. The pathologist may study the tissue under a microscope or perform other tests. When only a sample of tissue is removed, the procedure is called an incisional biopsy. When an entire lump or suspicious area is removed, the procedure is called an excisional biopsy. When a sample of tissue or fluid is removed with a needle, the procedure is called a needle biopsy, core biopsy, or fine-needle aspiration.

Bone marrow: The soft, sponge-like tissue in the center of most large bones. It produces white blood cells, red blood cells, and platelets.

Brachytherapy (BRAKE-ih-THER-a-pee): A procedure in which radioactive material sealed in needles, seeds, wires, or catheters is placed directly into or near a tumor. Also called internal radiation, implant radiation, or interstitial radiation therapy.

Cancer: A term for diseases in which abnormal cells divide without control. Cancer cells can invade nearby tissues and can spread through the bloodstream and lymphatic system to other parts of the body. There are several main types of cancer. Carcinoma is cancer that begins in the skin or in tissues that line or cover internal organs. Sarcoma is cancer that begins in bone, cartilage, fat, muscle, blood vessels, or other connective or supportive tissue. Leukemia is cancer that starts in blood-forming tissue such as the bone marrow, and causes large numbers of abnormal blood cells to be produced and enter the bloodstream.

Lymphoma and multiple myeloma are cancers that begin in the cells of the immune system.

Cell: The individual unit that makes up the tissues of the body. All living things are made up of one or more cells.

Chemotherapy (kee-mo-THER-a-pee): Treatment with drugs that kill cancer.

Clinical trial: A type of research study that tests how well new medical interventions work in people. Such studies test new methods of screening, prevention, diagnosis, or treatment of a disease. Studies may be carried out in a clinic or other medical facility. Also called a clinical study.

Colonoscopy (ko-lun-AHS-ko-pee): An examination of the inside of the colon using a thin, lighted tube (called a colonoscope) inserted into the rectum. If abnormal areas are seen, tissue can be removed and examined under a microscope to determine whether disease is present.

Complementary and alternative medicine: CAM. Forms of treatment that are used in addition to (complementary) or instead of (alternative) standard treatments. These practices generally are not considered standard medical approaches. Standard treatments have gone through a long and careful research process to prove they are safe and effective, but less is known about CAM. CAM may include dietary supplements, megadose vitamins, herbal preparations, special teas, acupuncture, massage therapy, magnet therapy, spiritual healing, and meditation.

CT scan: Computed tomography scan. A series of detailed pictures of areas inside the body taken from different angles; the pictures are created by a computer linked to an x-ray machine. Also called computerized tomography and computerized axial tomography (CAT) scan.

Diethylstilbestrol (dye-ETH-ul-stil-BES-trol): DES.

A synthetic form of the hormone estrogen that was prescribed to pregnant women between about 1940 and 1971 because it was thought to prevent miscarriages.

DES may increase the risk of uterine, ovarian, or breast cancer in women who took it. DES also has been linked to an increased risk of clear cell carcinoma of the vagina or cervix in daughters exposed to DES before birth.

Dietitian: A health professional with special training in nutrition who can help with dietary choices. Also called a nutritionist.

Digestive tract (dye-JES-tiv): The organs through which food and liquids pass when they are swallowed, digested, and eliminated. These organs are the mouth, esophagus, stomach, small and large intestines, and rectum.

Digital rectal exam: DRE. An examination in which a doctor inserts a lubricated, gloved finger into the rectum to feel for abnormalities.

Double-contrast barium enema: A procedure in which x-rays of the colon and rectum are taken after a liquid containing barium is put into the rectum. Barium is a silver-white metallic compound that outlines the colon and rectum on an x-ray and helps show abnormalities. Air is put into the rectum and colon to further enhance the x-ray.

Epstein-Barr virus: EBV. A common virus that remains dormant in most people. It has been associated with certain cancers, including Burkitt's lymphoma, immunoblastic lymphoma, and nasopharyngeal carcinoma.

Estrogen (ES-tro-jin): A hormone that promotes the development and maintenance of female sex characteristics.

Excisional biopsy (ek-SI-zhun-al BY-op-see):

A surgical procedure in which an entire lump or suspicious area is removed for diagnosis. The tissue is then examined under a microscope.

External radiation (ray-dee-AY-shun): Radiation therapy that uses a machine to aim high-energy rays at the cancer. Also called external-beam radiation.

Fecal occult blood test (FEE-kul o-KULT): FOBT.

A test to check for blood in stool. (Fecal refers to stool; occult means hidden.)

Fertility (fer-TIL-i-tee): The ability to produce children.

Gene: The functional and physical unit of heredity passed from parent to offspring. Genes are pieces of DNA, and most genes contain the information for making a specific protein.

Genetic testing: Analyzing DNA to look for a genetic alteration that may indicate an increased risk for developing a specific disease or disorder.

Helicobacter pylori (HEEL-ih-ko-BAK-ter pye-LOR-ee): H. pylori. Bacteria that cause inflammation and ulcers in the stomach and small intestine.

Hematologist (hee-ma-TOL-o-jist): A doctor who specializes in treating blood disorders.

Hepatitis B virus: A virus that causes hepatitis (inflammation of the liver). It is carried and passed to others through blood or sexual contact. Also, infants born to infected mothers may become infected with the virus.

Hepatitis C virus: A virus that causes hepatitis (inflammation of the liver). It is carried and passed to others through blood or sexual contact. Also, infants born to infected mothers may become infected with the virus.

Hormone: A chemical made by glands in the body. Hormones circulate in the bloodstream and control the actions of certain cells or organs. Some hormones can also be made in a laboratory.

Hormone therapy: Treatment that adds, blocks, or removes hormones. For certain conditions (such as diabetes or menopause), hormones are given to adjust low hormone levels. To slow or stop the growth of certain cancers (such as prostate and breast cancer), hormones may be given to block the body's natural hormones. Sometimes surgery is needed to remove the gland that makes hormones. Also called hormonal therapy, hormone treatment, or endocrine therapy.

Human herpesvirus 8: HHV8. A member of the herpes family of viruses. It is a risk factor for Kaposi's sarcoma, a rare cancer that can cause skin lesions.

Human immunodeficiency virus: HIV. The cause of acquired immunodeficiency syndrome (AIDS).

Human papillomavirus (pap-ih-LO-ma-VYE-rus): HPV. A virus that causes abnormal tissue growth (warts) and is associated with some types of cancer.

Human T-cell leukemia virus type 1: A retrovirus that infects T cells (a type of white blood cell) and can cause leukemia and lymphoma. HTLV-1 is spread by sharing syringes or needles used to inject drugs, through sexual contact, and from mother to child at birth or through breast-feeding.

Imaging procedure: A method of producing pictures of areas inside the body.

Implant radiation (ray-dee-AY-shun): A procedure in which radioactive material sealed in needles, seeds, wires, or catheters is placed directly into or near a tumor. Also called brachytherapy, internal radiation, or interstitial radiation.

Incisional biopsy (in-SIH-zhun-al BY-op-see): A surgical procedure in which a portion of a lump or suspicious area is removed for diagnosis. The tissue is then examined under a microscope.

Infection: Invasion and multiplication of germs in the body. Infections can occur in any part of the body, and can spread throughout the body. The germs may be bacteria, viruses, yeast, or fungi. They can cause a fever and other problems, depending on where the infection occurs. When the body's natural defense system is strong, it can often fight the germs and prevent infection. Cancer treatment can weaken the natural defense system.

Infertility: The inability to produce children.

Internal radiation (ray-dee-AY-shun): A procedure in which radioactive material sealed in needles, seeds, wires, or catheters is placed directly into or near a tumor. Also called brachytherapy, implant radiation, or interstitial radiation therapy.

Ionizing radiation (EYE-ah-NIZE-ing ray-dee-AY- shun): A type of high-frequency radiation produced by x-ray procedures, radioactive substances, rays that enter the Earth's atmosphere from outer space, and other sources. Ionizing radiation can enter cells and lead to health risks, including cancer, at certain doses.

Leukemia (loo-KEE-mee-a): Cancer that starts in blood-forming tissue such as the bone marrow, and causes large numbers of blood cells to be produced and enter the bloodstream.

Leukocyte (LOO-ko-site): A white blood cell. Refers to a blood cell that does not contain hemoglobin. White blood cells include lymphocytes, neutrophils, eosinophils, macrophages, and mast cells. These cells are made by bone marrow and help the body fight infection and other diseases.

Local therapy: Treatment that affects cells in the tumor and the area close to it.

Lymph node (limf node): A rounded mass of lymphatic tissue that is surrounded by a capsule of connective tissue. Lymph nodes filter lymph (lymphatic fluid), and they store lymphocytes (white blood cells). They are located along lymphatic vessels. Also called a lymph gland.

Lymphatic system (lim-FAT-ik SIS-tem): The tissues and organs that produce, store, and carry white blood cells that fight infections and other diseases. This system includes the bone marrow, spleen, thymus, lymph nodes, and lymphatic vessels (a network of thin tubes that carry lymph and white blood cells).

Lymphatic vessels branch, like blood vessels, into all the tissues of the body.

Lymphoma (lim-FO-ma): Cancer that begins in cells of the immune system.

Malignant (ma-LIG-nant): Cancerous. Malignant tumors can invade and destroy nearby tissue and spread to other parts of the body.

Mammogram (MAM-o-gram): An x-ray of the breast.

Medical oncologist (MED-i-kul on-KOL-o-jist): A doctor who specializes in diagnosing and treating cancer using chemotherapy, hormonal therapy, and biological therapy. A medical oncologist often is the main health care provider for someone who has cancer. A medical oncologist also provides supportive care and may coordinate treatment provided by other specialists.

Melanoma (MEL-ah-NO-ma): A form of skin cancer that arises in melanocytes, the cells that produce pigment. Melanoma usually begins in a mole.

Menopausal hormone therapy: Hormones (estrogen, progesterone, or both) given to women after menopause to replace the hormones no longer produced by the ovaries. Also called hormone replacement therapy or HRT.

Menopause (MEN-o-pawz): The time of life when a woman's menstrual periods stop permanently. Also called "change of life."

Metastasis (meh-TAS-ta-sis): The spread of cancer from one part of the body to another. A tumor formed by cells that have spread is called a "metastatic tumor" or a "metastasis." The metastatic tumor contains cells that are like those in the original (primary) tumor. The plural form of metastasis is metastases (meh-TAS-ta- seez).

Mole: A benign growth on the skin (usually tan, brown, or flesh-colored) that contains a cluster of melanocytes and surrounding supportive tissue.

MRI: Magnetic resonance imaging (mag-NET-ik REZ-o-nans IM-a-jing). A procedure in which radio

waves and a powerful magnet linked to a computer are used to create detailed pictures of areas inside the body. These pictures can show the difference between normal and diseased tissue. MRI makes better images of organs and soft tissue than other scanning techniques, such as CT or x-ray. MRI is especially useful for imaging the brain, spine, the soft tissue of joints, and the inside of bones. Also called nuclear magnetic resonance imaging.

Mutation: Any change in the DNA of a cell. Mutations may be caused by mistakes during cell division, or they may be caused by exposure to DNA-damaging agents in the environment. Mutations can be harmful, beneficial, or have no effect. If they occur in cells that make eggs or sperm, they can be inherited; if mutations occur in other types of cells, they are not inherited.

Certain mutations may lead to cancer or other diseases.

Organ: A part of the body that performs a specific function. For example, the heart is an organ.

Pap test: The collection of cells from the cervix for examination under a microscope. It is used to detect cancer and changes that may lead to cancer. Also called a Pap smear.

Pathologist (pa-THOL-o-jist): A doctor who identifies diseases by studying cells and tissues under a microscope.

PET scan: Positron emission tomography scan. A procedure in which a small amount of radioactive glucose (sugar) is injected into a vein, and a scanner is used to make detailed, computerized pictures of areas inside the body where the glucose is used. Because cancer cells often use more glucose than normal cells, the pictures can be used to find cancer cells in the body.

Polyp (POL-ip): A growth that protrudes from a mucous membrane.

Primary tumor: The original tumor.

Progestin (pro-JES-tin): Any natural or laboratory- made substance that has some or all of the biologic effects of progesterone, a female hormone.

Quality of life: The overall enjoyment of life. Many clinical trials assess the effects of cancer and its treatment on the quality of life. These studies measure aspects of an individual's sense of well-being and ability to carry out various activities.

Radiation oncologist (ray-dee-AY-shun on-KOL-o-jist): A doctor who specializes in using radiation to treat cancer.

Radiation therapy (ray-dee-AY-shun THER-ah-pee): The use of high-energy radiation from x-rays, gamma rays, neutrons, and other sources to kill cancer cells and shrink tumors. Radiation may come from a machine outside the body (external-beam radiation therapy), or it may come from radioactive material placed in the body near cancer cells (internal radiation therapy, implant radiation, or brachytherapy). Systemic radiation therapy uses a radioactive substance, such as a radiolabeled monoclonal antibody, that circulates throughout the body. Also called radiotherapy.

Radioactive: (RAY-dee-o-AK-tiv): Giving off radiation.

Radioactive fallout (RAY-dee-o-AK-tiv): Airborne radioactive particles that fall to the ground during and after an atomic bombing, nuclear weapons test, or nuclear plant accident.

Radionuclide scan (RAY-dee-o-NEW-klide): A test that produces pictures (scans) of internal parts of the body. The person is given an injection or swallows a small amount of radioactive material; a machine called a scanner then measures the radioactivity in certain organs.

Radon (RAY-don): A radioactive gas that is released by uranium, a substance found in soil and rock. Breathing in too much radon can damage lung cells and lead to lung cancer.

Recurrence: The return of cancer, at the same place as the original (primary) tumor or in another location, after the tumor had disappeared.

Risk factor: Something that may increase the chance of developing a disease. Some examples of risk factors for cancer include age, a family history of certain cancers, use of tobacco products, certain eating habits, obesity, exposure to radiation or other cancer-causing agents, and certain genetic changes.

Screening: Checking for disease when there are no symptoms.

Side effect: A problem that occurs when treatment affects healthy tissues or organs. Some common side effects of cancer treatment are fatigue, pain, nausea, vomiting, decreased blood cell counts, hair loss, and mouth sores.

Sigmoidoscopy (sig-moid-OSS-ko-pee): Inspection of the lower colon using a thin, lighted tube called a sigmoidoscope. Samples of tissue or cells may be collected for examination under a microscope. Also called proctosigmoidoscopy.

Sonogram (SAHN-o-gram): A computer picture of areas inside the body created by bouncing high-energy sound waves (ultrasound) off internal tissues or organs. Also called an ultrasonogram.

Spiral CT scan: A detailed picture of areas inside the body. The pictures are created by a computer linked to an x-ray machine that scans the body in a spiral path. Also called helical computed tomography.

Stage: The extent of a cancer within the body. Staging it based on the size of the tumor, whether lymph nodes contain cancer, and whether the disease has spread from the original site to other parts of the body.

Stem cell: A cell from which other types of cells develop. Blood cells develop from blood-forming stem cells.

Stem cell transplantation: A method of replacing immature blood-forming cells that were destroyed by cancer treatment. The stem cells are given to the person after treatment to help the bone marrow recover and continue producing healthy blood cells.

Supportive care: Care given to improve the quality of life of patients who have a serious or life-threatening disease. The goal of supportive care is to prevent or treat as early as possible the symptoms of the disease, side effects caused by treatment of the disease, and psychological, social, and spiritual problems related to the disease or its treatment. Also called palliative care, comfort care, and symptom management.

Surgeon: A doctor who removes or repairs a part of the body by operating on the patient.

Surgery (SER-juh-ree): A procedure to remove or repair a part of the body or to find out whether disease is present. An operation.

Symptom: An indication that a person has a condition or disease. Some examples of symptoms are headache, fever, fatigue, nausea, vomiting, and pain.

Systemic therapy (sis-TEM-ik THER-a-pee): Treatment using substances that travel through the bloodstream, reaching and affecting cells all over the body.

Thyroid (THIGH-royd): A gland located beneath the voice box (larynx) that produces thyroid hormone. The thyroid helps regulate growth and metabolism.

Tissue (TIH-shoo): A group or layer of cells that are alike and that work together to perform a specific function.

Tumor (TOO-mer): A mass of excess tissue that results from abnormal cell division. Tumors perform no useful body function. They may be benign (not cancerous) or malignant (cancerous).

Tumor marker: A substance sometimes found in the blood, other body fluids, or tissues. A high level of tumor marker may mean that a certain type of cancer is in the body. Examples of tumor markers include

CA 125 (ovarian cancer), CA 15-3 (breast cancer), CEA (ovarian, lung, breast, pancreas, and gastrointestinal tract cancers), and PSA (prostate cancer). Also called biomarker.

Ultrasound: A procedure in which high-energy sound waves (ultrasound) are bounced off internal tissues or organs and make echoes. The echo patterns are shown on the screen of an ultrasound machine, forming a picture of body tissues called a sonogram. Also called ultrasonography.

Ultraviolet radiation (ul-tra-VYE-o-let ray-dee-AY-shun): UV radiation. Invisible rays that are part of the energy that comes from the sun. UV radiation also comes from sun lamps and tanning beds. UV radiation can damage the skin and cause melanoma and other types of skin cancer. UV radiation that reaches the Earth's surface is made up of two types of rays, called UVA and UVB rays. UVB rays are more likely than UVA rays to cause sunburn, but UVA rays pass deeper into the skin. Scientists have long thought that UVB radiation can cause melanoma and other types of skin cancer. They now think that UVA radiation also may add to skin damage that can lead to skin cancer and cause premature aging. For this reason, skin specialists recommend that people use sunscreens that reflect, absorb, or scatter both kinds of UV radiation.

Virtual colonoscopy (ko-lun-AHS-ko-pee): A method under study to examine the colon by taking a series of x-rays (called a CT scan) and using a high-powered computer to reconstruct 2-D and 3-D pictures of the interior surfaces of the colon from these x-rays. The pictures can be saved, manipulated to better viewing angles, and reviewed after the procedure, even years later. Also called computed tomography colography.

Virus (VYE-rus): A microorganism that can infect cells and cause disease.

X-ray: A type of high-energy radiation. In low doses, x-rays are used to diagnose diseases by making pictures of the inside of the body. In high doses, x-rays are used to treat cancer.

ABOUT THE AUTHOR

Keith Garner, M.D is a specialist oncologist and he has been at the forefront of cancer research, prevention, and treatment. He has also done a lot of work in cancer enlightenment and has lead a lot of outreach campaigns to educate people about cancer.

He is married and lives with his wife and their 3 kids. When he is not working or volunteering, he loves to go fishing and hiking with his family.